# GOOD ENERGY:

---

## Unlocking the Secrets to Optimal Health and Vitality

### By CHARLES HARRISON, MD

# *Dedication*

To all those who seek to understand and optimize their health,

To the tireless researchers and healthcare professionals working to uncover the mysteries of human wellness,

To my family and friends, whose unwavering support and love inspire me every day,

And to every reader embarking on this journey towards a healthier, more vibrant life—

This book is for you. May it serve as a beacon of hope, knowledge, and empowerment on your path to well-being.

# TABLE OF CONTENTS

## Understanding Metabolic Health: The Key to Longevity and Wellbeing

### The Hidden Root Cause of Modern Health Issues

In the modern world, we are witnessing an alarming rise in chronic health conditions such as depression, anxiety, infertility, insomnia, heart disease, erectile dysfunction, type 2 diabetes, Alzheimer's, dementia, and cancer. These illnesses not only diminish our quality of life but also shorten our lifespan. Despite advancements in medical technology and healthcare, these conditions continue to proliferate at an unprecedented rate. The question that perplexes both scientists and medical professionals alike is: Why?

The answer lies hidden in the very core of our biology, within the tiny powerhouses of our cells known as mitochondria. These microscopic organelles are responsible for producing the energy our cells need to function optimally. This process, known as cellular respiration, is the cornerstone of our metabolic health. When our cells produce energy efficiently, our bodies thrive; when this process falters, a cascade of health issues ensues.

## Metabolic Dysfunction: The Common Denominator

At the heart of nearly every chronic illness is a common root cause: metabolic dysfunction. Our bodies use the process of metabolism to turn the food we ingest into energy. It is a complex system involving hormones, enzymes, and numerous biochemical reactions. When this system works well, it powers everything from our heartbeat to our thoughts. However, when it goes awry, it sets the stage for a myriad of health problems.

Metabolic dysfunction occurs when our cells become inefficient at producing energy. This inefficiency can stem from various factors, including poor diet, lack of exercise, inadequate sleep, chronic stress, and environmental toxins. When our cells cannot produce enough energy, they cannot perform their functions properly, leading to cellular damage, inflammation, and ultimately, disease.

## The Role of Inflammation and Insulin Resistance

Two key players in the development of metabolic dysfunction are chronic inflammation and insulin resistance. Inflammation is the body's natural response to injury or infection, but when it becomes chronic, it can cause harm. Persistent inflammation can damage tissues and organs, leading to diseases such as heart disease, type 2 diabetes, and Alzheimer's.

Insulin resistance, on the other hand, occurs when our cells become less responsive to insulin, a hormone that helps regulate blood sugar levels. This condition forces the pancreas to produce more insulin to compensate, which can eventually lead to type 2 diabetes and other metabolic disorders. Insulin resistance is also closely linked to obesity, another major risk factor for chronic diseases.

## Environmental and Lifestyle Factors

The modern lifestyle is a breeding ground for metabolic dysfunction. Our diets are often high in processed foods, sugars, and unhealthy fats, which can lead to poor metabolic health. Sedentary lifestyles, characterized by long hours of sitting and minimal physical activity, exacerbate the problem. Additionally, chronic stress and poor sleep quality disrupt hormonal balance and circadian rhythms, further impairing metabolic function.

Environmental toxins also play a significant role. Chemicals found in plastics, pesticides, and pollution can interfere with our endocrine system and disrupt metabolic processes. These toxins accumulate in our bodies over time, contributing to chronic inflammation and metabolic dysfunction.

## A New Approach to Health

Understanding that metabolic dysfunction is the hidden root cause of many modern health issues is a game-changer. It moves the emphasis from taking care of the symptoms to dealing with the underlying problem.

By optimizing our metabolic health, we can prevent and even reverse many chronic diseases.

This book aims to equip you with the knowledge and tools to take control of your metabolic health. We will explore practical strategies for improving diet, incorporating movement into daily life, managing stress, enhancing sleep quality, and minimizing exposure to environmental toxins. By making these changes, you can support your cells in producing good energy, thereby enhancing your overall health and wellbeing.

The path to good health is within reach. It starts with understanding the critical role of metabolism and taking proactive steps to nurture it. Welcome to the journey towards a healthier, more vibrant life.

## A New Vision for Optimal Health

Imagine a world where chronic diseases such as depression, anxiety, heart disease, type 2 diabetes, Alzheimer's, and cancer are rare rather than rampant. A world where vibrant health, boundless energy, and mental clarity are not just aspirations but everyday realities for people of all ages. This might seem like an unreachable ideal, but emerging scientific research and advancements in health technology are bringing this vision closer to reality. At the core of this transformation is a profound understanding of metabolic health.

## The Foundation of Optimal Health: Metabolic Function

Metabolism is the set of life-sustaining chemical reactions in our bodies that convert food into energy, which powers every cell, organ, and system. This fundamental process, often taken for granted, is the key to our overall health and longevity. Optimal metabolic function means that our cells are efficiently producing and using energy, leading to a state of balanced bodily functions and resilience against diseases.

### Understanding the Energy Equation

Energy is the currency of life. Every thought we think, every step we take, every beat of our heart depends on our cells' ability to produce energy. When our cells generate energy efficiently, we experience vitality and well-being. Conversely, when this process is compromised, we become susceptible to a host of health problems. This energy equation is crucial: good energy production equals good health; poor energy production equals poor health.

## The Paradigm Change: From Treating Symptoms to Addressing the Cause

For decades, healthcare has largely focused on managing symptoms rather than addressing the root causes of diseases. This approach has led to a fragmented understanding of health, where each symptom is treated as an isolated issue. However, groundbreaking research reveals that many chronic conditions share a common root cause: metabolic dysfunction. By shifting our focus to improving metabolic health, we can tackle these conditions at their source, leading to more effective and sustainable health outcomes.

## Personalized Health Through Technology

Advancements in health technology are revolutionizing how we approach and understand our bodies. Wearable devices and affordable diagnostic tools now allow us to monitor critical biomarkers related to metabolic health, such as glucose levels, heart rate variability, and inflammation markers. These technologies provide real-time feedback, empowering individuals to make informed decisions about their health.

With these tools, we can adopt a proactive approach to health, catching early signs of metabolic dysfunction before they develop into serious diseases. This personalized health monitoring represents a significant shift from reactive to preventive healthcare, enabling us to maintain optimal health throughout our lives.

## Holistic Lifestyle Strategies

Achieving optimal metabolic health requires a holistic approach that encompasses diet, exercise, sleep, and stress management. Here are some key strategies:

**Nutrition:** Simplify your diet by focusing on whole, unprocessed foods. Implementing six lifelong food principles—such as reducing sugar intake, eating a variety of colorful vegetables, and balancing macronutrients—can profoundly impact metabolic health.

**Movement:** Integrate simple, consistent physical activity into your daily routine. Exercise doesn't have to mean spending hours at the gym; even small changes like taking the stairs, walking more, and incorporating short bursts of activity can boost metabolic function.

**Sleep:** Prioritize sleep by maintaining a regular sleep schedule, creating a restful environment, and addressing any sleep disorders. Quality sleep is essential for metabolic regulation and overall health.

**Stress Management:** Practice mindfulness, meditation, and other stress-reduction techniques to lower chronic stress levels. Chronic stress can disrupt metabolic processes and lead to inflammation and insulin resistance.

**Environmental Exposure:** Utilize the benefits of cold and heat exposure through practices like cold showers, saunas, or controlled heat exposure, which can improve metabolic resilience and overall health.

**Empowering Your Health Journey**

There is no one-size-fits-all approach to achieving good health. It requires a personalized approach, informed by an understanding of your unique metabolic profile and lifestyle. This book will guide you through actionable steps to monitor, understand, and improve your metabolic health, offering practical advice and insights grounded in the latest scientific research.

By embracing this new vision for optimal health, you are not just aiming to prevent disease; you are striving to enhance your quality of life, boost your energy levels, and achieve a state of holistic well-being. It's time to take control of your health journey, harness the power of your metabolism, and live a life filled with good energy. Welcome to the future of health.

## Overview of Metabolic Function and Its Impact

At the heart of our health and vitality lies a process that often goes unnoticed: metabolism. This intricate set of chemical reactions occurring within our cells is the cornerstone of our overall health. Understanding metabolic function is crucial because it directly influences how our bodies generate and use energy, which in turn affects every aspect of our physical and mental well-being.

### What is Metabolism?

Metabolism encompasses all the biochemical processes that occur within our bodies to maintain life. These processes can be broadly divided into two categories: catabolism and anabolism.

**Catabolism:** This is the process of breaking down molecules to produce energy. For instance, when we eat, our bodies break down carbohydrates, fats, and proteins into smaller molecules like glucose, fatty acids, and amino acids. These molecules are then used to produce adenosine triphosphate (ATP), the primary energy currency of cells.

**Anabolism:** This is the process of building up complex molecules from simpler ones, utilizing the energy produced during catabolism. Anabolic processes are responsible for the growth and repair of tissues, the synthesis of hormones, and the storage of energy for future use.

### The Role of Mitochondria

Central to the process of metabolism are mitochondria, the "powerhouses" of our cells. These organelles are where most of the ATP is produced through a process called oxidative phosphorylation. The efficiency of mitochondrial function is a key determinant of metabolic health. When mitochondria are functioning optimally, they produce ample energy with minimal waste. However, when they are compromised, it leads to insufficient energy production and an increase in harmful byproducts, such as reactive oxygen species (ROS), which can damage cells and tissues.

### Key Components of Metabolic Function

Several key components contribute to overall metabolic function:

**Glucose Metabolism:** Glucose, derived from carbohydrates, is a primary energy source. It is metabolized through glycolysis and the Krebs cycle to produce ATP. Insulin, a hormone produced by the pancreas, plays a critical role in regulating glucose levels in the blood by facilitating its uptake into cells.

**Lipid Metabolism:** Fats are broken down into fatty acids and glycerol, which can also be used to produce ATP. Additionally, fats are essential for the construction of cell membranes and the production of certain hormones.

**Protein Metabolism:** Proteins are broken down into amino acids, which can be used for energy production, but more importantly, are crucial for building and repairing tissues, and producing enzymes and hormones.

**Thermogenesis:** the mechanism by which the human body produces heat. It is a part of energy expenditure and involves both basal metabolic rate (the energy required for basic physiological functions) and the thermic effect of food (the energy used in digestion, absorption, and metabolism of food).

### Impact of Metabolic Function on Health

The efficiency of metabolic processes directly impacts our health in several ways:

**Energy Levels:** Proper metabolic function ensures that our cells produce sufficient energy, which translates to overall vitality and stamina. Poor metabolic health can lead to fatigue and reduced physical and mental performance.

**Weight Management:** Metabolism plays a significant role in determining how efficiently our bodies use and store energy. Disruptions in metabolic processes can lead to weight gain or difficulty losing weight, contributing to obesity and related health issues.

**Chronic Diseases:** Metabolic dysfunction is at the root of many chronic conditions, including type 2 diabetes, cardiovascular diseases, and certain cancers. For example, insulin resistance, a hallmark of metabolic dysfunction, is a major risk factor for type 2 diabetes and heart disease.

**Mental Health:** There is a strong link between metabolic health and mental well-being. Conditions like depression and anxiety have been associated with metabolic dysfunction, likely due to the impact of metabolic health on brain function and inflammation.

**Aging:** Efficient metabolic function can slow down the aging process by reducing cellular damage and improving the repair mechanisms of cells. Conversely, metabolic dysfunction accelerates aging and increases susceptibility to age-related diseases.

## Optimizing Metabolic Health

Given its profound impact on overall health, optimizing metabolic function should be a primary goal. This can be achieved through:

**Balanced Nutrition:** Consuming a diet rich in whole, unprocessed foods, with balanced macronutrients and adequate micronutrients, supports metabolic health.

**Regular Physical Activity:** Exercise enhances mitochondrial function, improves insulin sensitivity, and supports overall metabolic processes.

**Quality Sleep:** Adequate and quality sleep is essential for the regulation of metabolic processes and hormonal balance.

**Stress Management:** Chronic stress negatively impacts metabolism by disrupting hormonal balance and promoting inflammation. Mindfulness, meditation, and relaxation techniques can help manage stress.

**Environmental Factors:** Minimizing exposure to environmental toxins and incorporating practices like cold and heat exposure can enhance metabolic resilience.

# CHAPTER 1: THE POWER OF METABOLIC HEALTH

## The Science of Energy: How Our Cells Create and Use Fuel

### Cellular Energy Production Explained

At the core of our health and vitality lies the process by which our cells produce energy. This intricate process, essential for all biological functions, takes place within the mitochondria, often referred to as the powerhouses of the cell. Understanding cellular energy production is crucial for grasping how our bodies operate and maintain health. This chapter delves into the details of how our cells convert nutrients into usable energy, the role of mitochondria, and the impact of this process on overall health.

### The Basics of Cellular Energy Production

Cellular energy production primarily revolves around the molecule adenosine triphosphate (ATP). ATP is the energy currency of the cell, providing the energy necessary for various cellular processes, including muscle contraction, nerve impulse propagation, and chemical synthesis. The production of ATP occurs through several interconnected pathways, the most significant of which are glycolysis, the citric acid cycle (Krebs cycle), and oxidative phosphorylation.

## Glycolysis: The First Step

Glycolysis is the initial stage of glucose metabolism and occurs in the cytoplasm of the cell. This process breaks down one molecule of glucose (a six-carbon sugar) into two molecules of pyruvate (a three-carbon compound). Glycolysis produces a net gain of two ATP molecules and two molecules of nicotinamide adenine dinucleotide (NADH), a carrier of electrons used in further stages of energy production.

## The Citric Acid Cycle: Harvesting Electrons

The pyruvate molecules produced during glycolysis are transported into the mitochondria, where they are converted into acetyl-CoA, the starting molecule for the citric acid cycle (also known as the Krebs cycle or TCA cycle). The citric acid cycle takes place in the mitochondrial matrix and involves a series of enzyme-catalyzed reactions that further break down acetyl-CoA into carbon dioxide and high-energy electron carriers: NADH and flavin adenine dinucleotide ($FADH_2$).

For each acetyl-CoA molecule that enters the cycle, the citric acid cycle produces:

Two molecules of carbon dioxide

Three molecules of NADH

One molecule of $FADH_2$

One molecule of ATP (or GTP, which is converted to ATP)

The NADH and FADH2 produced are crucial for the next stage of cellular respiration: oxidative phosphorylation.

## Oxidative Phosphorylation: The Powerhouse of Energy Production

Oxidative phosphorylation, which occurs in the inner mitochondrial membrane, is the final and most productive stage of cellular respiration. This process involves the electron transport chain (ETC) and ATP synthase, a complex enzyme that synthesizes ATP.

**Electron Transport Chain (ETC):** The ETC is a series of protein complexes embedded in the inner mitochondrial membrane. Electrons from NADH and FADH2 are transferred through these complexes, releasing energy at each step. This energy is used to pump protons (H+) from the mitochondrial matrix into the intermembrane space, creating an electrochemical gradient known as the proton motive force.

**ATP Synthase:** The proton motive force drives protons back into the mitochondrial matrix through ATP synthase. As protons flow through ATP synthase, it catalyzes the conversion of adenosine diphosphate (ADP) and inorganic phosphate (Pi) into ATP. This process, called chemiosmosis, produces the majority of ATP in cellular respiration—approximately 30-34 ATP molecules per glucose molecule.

**The Role of Mitochondria**

Mitochondria are unique organelles with their own DNA, capable of dividing and increasing in number within a cell. They are the primary site of ATP production through oxidative phosphorylation and are also involved in other critical cellular processes such as apoptosis (programmed cell death), calcium storage, and the generation of reactive oxygen species (ROS).

**The Impact on Health**

Efficient cellular energy production is vital for maintaining health and preventing disease. When mitochondria function optimally, they produce sufficient energy with minimal harmful byproducts. However, when mitochondrial function is compromised, several adverse effects can occur:

**Energy Deficiency:** Insufficient ATP production can lead to fatigue, muscle weakness, and impaired organ function. This is often seen in mitochondrial disorders and chronic fatigue syndrome.

**Oxidative Stress:** The electron transport chain can leak electrons, which combine with oxygen to form reactive oxygen species (ROS). Excessive ROS can damage cellular components, leading to oxidative stress, inflammation, and aging. Antioxidant defenses typically neutralize ROS, but chronic metabolic dysfunction can overwhelm these defenses.

**Metabolic Diseases:** Mitochondrial dysfunction is linked to various metabolic diseases, including obesity, type 2 diabetes, cardiovascular diseases, and neurodegenerative disorders like Alzheimer's and Parkinson's diseases. These conditions often involve impaired energy metabolism and increased oxidative stress.

## Optimizing Cellular Energy Production

Enhancing mitochondrial function and cellular energy production is key to improving overall health. Here are some strategies:

**Balanced Nutrition:** Consuming a diet rich in whole, unprocessed foods provides the necessary nutrients for efficient cellular respiration. Nutrients such as coenzyme Q10, magnesium, and B vitamins are vital for mitochondrial function.

**Regular Exercise:** Physical activity boosts mitochondrial biogenesis (the creation of new mitochondria) and enhances their efficiency. Both aerobic exercises, like running and cycling, and resistance training, like weightlifting, are beneficial.

**Quality Sleep:** Adequate sleep supports mitochondrial repair and regeneration. Poor sleep quality can disrupt mitochondrial function and energy production.

**Stress Management:** Chronic stress impairs mitochondrial function. Techniques like mindfulness, meditation, and yoga can help manage stress levels.

**Environmental Exposure:** Controlled exposure to cold and heat (e.g., cold showers, saunas) can stimulate mitochondrial activity and improve resilience.

By understanding and optimizing cellular energy production, we can enhance our vitality, prevent disease, and improve our quality of life. This foundational knowledge empowers us to take proactive steps toward achieving and maintaining optimal health.

## The Connection Between Metabolic Function and Chronic Diseases

The rising prevalence of chronic diseases such as type 2 diabetes, heart disease, Alzheimer's, cancer, and depression poses a significant challenge to global health. A growing body of research points to a common underlying factor in many of these conditions: metabolic dysfunction. Metabolic health is crucial for maintaining the optimal function of our cells, and disruptions in this complex system can lead to a wide range of chronic illnesses. This chapter explores the intricate relationship between metabolic function and chronic diseases, shedding light on how improving metabolic health can help prevent and manage these conditions.

### Metabolic Dysfunction: The Common Denominator

Metabolic dysfunction occurs when the body's processes for generating and using energy are impaired. This can result from various factors, including poor diet, lack of physical activity, inadequate sleep, chronic stress, and exposure to environmental toxins. At the cellular level, metabolic dysfunction often involves issues with mitochondrial function, insulin resistance, chronic inflammation, and oxidative stress.

## Insulin Resistance and Type 2 Diabetes

One of the most well-known connections between metabolic dysfunction and chronic disease is insulin resistance, a condition where cells become less responsive to insulin. Insulin is a hormone that helps regulate blood glucose levels by facilitating the uptake of glucose into cells for energy production. When cells resist insulin's effects, glucose builds up in the blood, leading to hyperglycemia.

Type 2 Diabetes: Chronic insulin resistance can lead to type 2 diabetes, characterized by high blood sugar levels and impaired glucose metabolism. Over time, high blood sugar can damage blood vessels, nerves, and organs, leading to complications such as cardiovascular disease, kidney failure, and neuropathy.

## Cardiovascular Diseases

Metabolic dysfunction is a significant risk factor for cardiovascular diseases (CVD), which include conditions like coronary artery disease, stroke, and hypertension. Key metabolic contributors to CVD include:

**Dyslipidemia:** Imbalances in lipid metabolism, such as elevated levels of low-density lipoprotein (LDL) cholesterol and triglycerides, and low levels of high-density lipoprotein (HDL) cholesterol, contribute to the formation of atherosclerotic plaques. These plaques can narrow and harden the arteries, increasing the risk of heart attack and stroke.

**Hypertension:** Insulin resistance and hyperinsulinemia (elevated insulin levels) can lead to hypertension, or high blood pressure. Insulin resistance can cause the kidneys to retain more sodium and water, increasing blood volume and pressure. Additionally, it can lead to endothelial dysfunction, reducing the elasticity of blood vessels and increasing resistance to blood flow.

**Inflammation:** Chronic inflammation, often associated with metabolic dysfunction, plays a central role in the development of atherosclerosis. Inflammatory markers such as C-reactive protein (CRP) are elevated in individuals with metabolic syndrome and are predictors of cardiovascular events.

### Neurodegenerative Diseases

Emerging evidence suggests a strong link between metabolic dysfunction and neurodegenerative diseases, including Alzheimer's and Parkinson's diseases.

**Alzheimer's Disease:** Often referred to as "type 3 diabetes," Alzheimer's disease has been linked to insulin resistance in the brain. Impaired insulin signaling can lead to reduced glucose uptake and energy production in neurons, contributing to cognitive decline and the accumulation of amyloid-beta plaques and tau tangles, hallmark features of Alzheimer's.

**Parkinson's Disease:** Mitochondrial dysfunction and oxidative stress are central to the pathogenesis of Parkinson's disease. The loss of mitochondrial function in dopaminergic neurons leads to energy deficits and increased vulnerability to oxidative damage, contributing to neurodegeneration.

**Cancer**

Metabolic dysfunction is also implicated in the development and progression of cancer. Cancer cells have altered metabolism, often characterized by increased glucose uptake and fermentation of glucose to lactate, even in the presence of oxygen (the Warburg effect).

**Cell Proliferation:** The altered metabolic state of cancer cells supports rapid cell proliferation by providing the necessary energy and biosynthetic precursors. Insulin resistance and hyperinsulinemia can promote cancer growth by increasing the levels of insulin-like growth factors (IGFs), which stimulate cell division and inhibit apoptosis.

**Obesity:** Obesity, a common consequence of metabolic dysfunction, is a major risk factor for several types of cancer, including breast, colon, and pancreatic cancer. Adipose tissue secretes pro-inflammatory cytokines and hormones that can create a pro-tumorigenic environment.

## Mental Health Disorders

The connection between metabolic function and mental health is becoming increasingly recognized. Metabolic dysfunction can impact brain health through several mechanisms:

**Depression and Anxiety:** Chronic inflammation and insulin resistance have been linked to depression and anxiety. Inflammatory cytokines can affect neurotransmitter function and brain structure, contributing to mood disorders. Insulin resistance can also impair glucose uptake in the brain, affecting energy metabolism and cognitive function.

**Cognitive Decline:** Metabolic syndrome is associated with an increased risk of cognitive decline and dementia. Poor metabolic health can lead to vascular changes, neuroinflammation, and insulin resistance in the brain, all of which contribute to cognitive impairments.

## Strategies to Improve Metabolic Health

Given the profound impact of metabolic function on chronic diseases, optimizing metabolic health is crucial. Here are some strategies:

**Diet:** Adopting a diet rich in whole, unprocessed foods, including vegetables, fruits, lean proteins, and healthy fats, can improve insulin sensitivity and reduce inflammation. Avoiding refined sugars, processed foods, and trans fats is also beneficial.

**Exercise:** Regular physical activity enhances mitochondrial function, improves insulin sensitivity, and reduces inflammation. Both aerobic and resistance training are effective in promoting metabolic health.

**Sleep:** Ensuring adequate and quality sleep is essential for metabolic regulation. Poor sleep can disrupt hormonal balance and increase the risk of insulin resistance and inflammation.

**Stress Management:** Chronic stress negatively impacts metabolic health by promoting insulin resistance and inflammation. Techniques such as mindfulness, meditation, and yoga can help manage stress levels.

**Weight Management:** Maintaining a healthy weight through diet and exercise can improve metabolic health and reduce the risk of chronic diseases.

**Environmental Exposure:** Reducing exposure to environmental toxins and incorporating practices like cold and heat exposure can enhance metabolic resilience and overall health.

By addressing metabolic dysfunction and implementing these strategies, we can significantly reduce the risk of chronic diseases and improve overall health and longevity. Understanding and optimizing metabolic function is a powerful approach to preventing and managing the chronic conditions that plague modern society.

## Real-Life Stories of Transformation

Understanding the science behind metabolic health is crucial, but seeing its impact on real lives can be truly inspiring. This chapter shares powerful stories of individuals who have transformed their health and well-being by focusing on improving their metabolic function. These personal accounts highlight the profound changes that are possible when we take control of our metabolic health.

### Sarah's Journey: Overcoming Type 2 Diabetes

Sarah, a 52-year-old schoolteacher, had struggled with her weight and energy levels for years. Diagnosed with type 2 diabetes, she was on multiple medications and felt trapped in a cycle of poor health. Her blood sugar levels were poorly controlled, and she faced constant fatigue, making it difficult to keep up with her students and family responsibilities.

Sarah decided to take charge of her health after reading about the link between diet and metabolic function. She started by making small, sustainable changes to her diet, focusing on whole, unprocessed foods. She reduced her intake of refined sugars and carbohydrates, incorporating more vegetables, lean proteins, and healthy fats into her meals.

Alongside dietary changes, Sarah began walking daily and gradually increased her physical activity to include strength training exercises. She also prioritized sleep and started practicing mindfulness meditation to manage stress.

Within six months, Sarah experienced remarkable changes. She lost 30 pounds, her blood sugar levels normalized, and she was able to reduce her diabetes medications under her doctor's supervision. Sarah's energy levels soared, and she felt more vibrant and engaged in her life than she had in years.

## John's Story: Battling Depression with Metabolic Health

John, a 38-year-old software engineer, had been dealing with chronic depression and anxiety for most of his adult life. Despite trying various medications and therapies, he struggled to find relief and often felt hopeless.

A turning point came when John attended a health seminar where he learned about the connection between metabolic health and mental well-being. Intrigued, he decided to explore this further and made several lifestyle changes to improve his metabolic function.

John adopted a diet rich in anti-inflammatory foods, including fatty fish, leafy greens, nuts, and berries. He cut out processed foods and significantly reduced his sugar intake. He also began a regular exercise regimen that included both aerobic activities and yoga.

Recognizing the importance of sleep, John established a consistent sleep routine and created a sleep-friendly environment by minimizing screen time before bed and ensuring his bedroom was dark and cool. To manage stress, he practiced mindfulness meditation and deep breathing exercises.

Over the course of a year, John's mental health improved dramatically. His episodes of depression became less frequent and severe, and his anxiety levels decreased. John found that he could manage his symptoms more effectively and enjoyed a better quality of life.

## Maria's Triumph: Reversing PCOS and Infertility

Maria, a 30-year-old marketing professional, had been diagnosed with polycystic ovary syndrome (PCOS) and struggled with irregular periods and infertility. Despite trying various treatments, she faced numerous setbacks and felt increasingly discouraged.

After researching alternative approaches, Maria discovered the impact of metabolic health on hormonal balance and fertility. She decided to overhaul her lifestyle to improve her metabolic function.

Maria adopted a nutrient-dense diet, focusing on whole foods, including plenty of vegetables, lean proteins, and healthy fats. She eliminated processed foods, refined sugars, and trans fats from her diet. She also incorporated regular exercise, including both cardio and strength training, into her routine.

To support her hormonal health, Maria prioritized sleep and practiced stress-reduction techniques such as yoga and mindfulness meditation. She also sought support from a healthcare provider knowledgeable about metabolic health and PCOS.

Within a year, Maria's menstrual cycles became regular, and she experienced significant improvements in her overall health. To her delight, she conceived naturally and gave birth to a healthy baby girl. Maria's journey underscored the profound impact that metabolic health can have on reproductive health and overall well-being.

## David's Victory: Conquering Heart Disease

David, a 65-year-old retired engineer, had a history of heart disease. He had undergone bypass surgery and was on multiple medications to manage his condition. Despite these interventions, David continued to experience angina and felt limited in his daily activities.

Determined to improve his health, David learned about the relationship between metabolic function and cardiovascular health. He decided to make significant lifestyle changes to support his metabolic health.

David adopted a heart-healthy diet rich in fruits, vegetables, whole grains, lean proteins, and healthy fats. He reduced his intake of sodium and processed foods. Regular physical activity became a cornerstone of his routine, and he incorporated both aerobic exercises and strength training.

David also focused on improving his sleep quality and managing stress through meditation and spending time in nature. He worked closely with his healthcare team to monitor his progress and adjust his medications as needed.

Over two years, David experienced remarkable improvements in his heart health. His angina symptoms diminished, his cholesterol levels improved, and he was able to reduce some of his medications under medical guidance. David regained his energy and enjoyed a more active and fulfilling retirement.

# CHAPTER 2: BIOMARKERS AND TECHNOLOGY: UNLOCKING HEALTH SECRETS

## Monitoring Metabolic Health: Tools and Techniques

### The Five Key Biomarkers to Track

To optimize metabolic health and prevent chronic diseases, it is essential to monitor specific biomarkers that provide insights into how well our bodies are functioning. Biomarkers are measurable indicators of biological processes, and tracking them can help us identify early signs of metabolic dysfunction, allowing for timely interventions. This chapter outlines five key biomarkers that are crucial for assessing metabolic health and offers guidance on how to monitor and interpret them.

### 1. Blood Glucose Levels

**Importance:**

Blood glucose levels indicate how well your body manages sugar, a primary source of energy. Maintaining balanced blood glucose levels is critical for preventing metabolic diseases such as type 2 diabetes and managing overall metabolic health.

**How to Track:**

**1. Fasting Blood Glucose (FBG):** Measures blood sugar levels after an overnight fast. A normal FBG level is below 100 mg/dL.

**Haemoglobin A1c (HbA1c):** Analyses average levels of glucose in the blood during the previous 2-3 months. The typical HbA1c level is less than 5.7%.

**Continuous Glucose Monitoring (CGM):** Provides real-time glucose readings throughout the day, offering insights into how diet, exercise, and stress impact glucose levels.

**Interpretation:**

**Normal:** FBG < 100 mg/dL, HbA1c < 5.7%

**Prediabetes:** FBG 100-125 mg/dL, HbA1c 5.7-6.4%

**Diabetes:** FBG ≥ 126 mg/dL, HbA1c ≥ 6.5%

**2. Lipid Profile**

**Importance:**

A lipid profile measures the levels of fats in the blood, including cholesterol and triglycerides. These levels are crucial indicators of cardiovascular health and metabolic function.

**How to Track:**

**Total Cholesterol:** Should be below 200 mg/dL.

**Low-Density Lipoprotein (LDL) Cholesterol:** Known as "bad" cholesterol, should be below 100 mg/dL.

**High-Density Lipoprotein (HDL) Cholesterol:** Known as "good" cholesterol, should be above 40 mg/dL for men and above 50 mg/dL for women.

**Triglycerides:** Should be below 150 mg/dL.

**Interpretation:**

**Healthy Levels:** Total cholesterol < 200 mg/dL, LDL < 100 mg/dL, HDL > 40 mg/dL (men) / > 50 mg/dL (women), Triglycerides < 150 mg/dL

**Borderline High:** Total cholesterol 200-239 mg/dL, LDL 100-159 mg/dL, HDL 40-59 mg/dL (men) / 50-59 mg/dL (women), Triglycerides 150-199 mg/dL

**High:** Total cholesterol ≥ 240 mg/dL, LDL ≥ 160 mg/dL, HDL < 40 mg/dL (men) / < 50 mg/dL (women), Triglycerides ≥ 200 mg/dL

### 3. Inflammatory Markers

**Importance:**

Chronic inflammation is a key contributor to many metabolic and cardiovascular diseases. Tracking inflammatory markers can help detect and address underlying inflammation.

**How to Track:**

**C-Reactive Protein (CRP):** A general marker of inflammation. High-sensitivity CRP (hs-CRP) is used to assess the risk of cardiovascular disease.

**Interleukin-6 (IL-6) and Tumor Necrosis Factor-alpha (TNF-α):** Cytokines involved in systemic inflammation.

**Interpretation:**

**Normal CRP Levels:** < 1.0 mg/L

**Moderate Risk:** 1.0-3.0 mg/L

**High Risk:** > 3.0 mg/L

Elevated IL-6 and TNF-α levels indicate higher levels of inflammation and potential metabolic dysfunction.

## 4. Insulin Levels

**Importance:**

Insulin is a hormone that regulates blood glucose levels. Monitoring insulin levels can help detect insulin resistance, a precursor to type 2 diabetes and other metabolic disorders.

**How to Track:**

**Fasting Insulin Test:** Measures insulin levels after fasting overnight.

**Homeostatic Model Assessment of Insulin Resistance (HOMA-IR):** Calculates insulin resistance using fasting insulin and glucose levels.

**Interpretation:**

**Normal Fasting Insulin:** 2-20 µU/mL

**HOMA-IR:** A score below 1.0 indicates optimal insulin sensitivity, while a score above 2.9 indicates significant insulin resistance.

## 5. Body Composition

**Importance:**

Body composition, particularly the ratio of fat to lean muscle mass, is a critical indicator of metabolic health. Excess body fat, especially visceral fat, is associated with increased risk of metabolic diseases.

**How to Track:**

**Body Mass Index (BMI):** A general measure of body fat based on height and weight. Normal BMI is 18.5-24.9.

**Waist Circumference:** Measures abdominal fat. Ideal waist circumference is below 40 inches for men and below 35 inches for women.

**Body Fat Percentage:** Provides a more precise measurement of body composition.

**Interpretation:**

**Healthy BMI:** 18.5-24.9

**Overweight:** 25-29.9

**Obese:** ≥ 30

**Ideal Waist Circumference:** < 40 inches (men), < 35 inches (women)

**Optimal Body Fat Percentage:** Varies by age and gender, generally around 18-24% for men and 25-31% for women.

## Using Health Technology to "See Inside Your Body"

In the pursuit of optimal health, technology has emerged as a powerful ally, offering unprecedented opportunities to gain insights into our bodies and monitor key aspects of our health. From wearable devices to advanced imaging techniques, health technology enables us to "see inside our bodies" with remarkable clarity and precision. This chapter explores the innovative ways in which technology is revolutionizing healthcare, empowering individuals to take proactive steps towards improving their metabolic health and overall well-being.

### Wearable Health Trackers

Wearable health trackers, such as smartwatches and fitness bands, have become ubiquitous tools for monitoring various aspects of health and fitness in real-time. These devices use sensors to track metrics like heart rate, activity levels, sleep patterns, and even stress levels throughout the day.

**Benefits:**

**Continuous Monitoring:** Wearable trackers provide continuous data, allowing users to track their health metrics throughout the day and identify patterns or trends.

**Personalized Insights:** Many wearable devices offer personalized insights and recommendations based on individual data, helping users make informed decisions about their health behaviors.

**Motivation and Accountability:** The ability to set goals, track progress, and receive feedback in real-time can motivate users to adopt healthier habits and stay accountable to their health goals.

## Continuous Glucose Monitors (CGMs)

Continuous glucose monitors (CGMs) are devices used primarily by individuals with diabetes to track their blood glucose levels continuously throughout the day. CGMs consist of a small sensor inserted under the skin, which measures glucose levels in the interstitial fluid and transmits the data to a receiver or smartphone app.

**Benefits:**

**Real-Time Glucose Monitoring:** CGMs provide real-time data on blood glucose levels, enabling individuals with diabetes to make immediate adjustments to their diet, exercise, or insulin therapy as needed.

**Trend Analysis:** CGM data can reveal trends in blood sugar levels, such as post-meal spikes or overnight lows, helping users understand how their lifestyle choices impact their glucose levels over time.

**Early Detection of Hypo- and Hyperglycemia:** CGMs can alert users to impending hypoglycemic (low blood sugar) or hyperglycemic (high blood sugar) events, allowing for early intervention to prevent complications.

**Body Composition Analyzers**

Body composition analyzers use advanced technology, such as bioelectrical impedance analysis (BIA) or dual-energy X-ray absorptiometry (DEXA), to assess body composition by measuring the distribution of fat, lean muscle, and bone mass in the body.

**Benefits:**

**Comprehensive Assessment:** Body composition analyzers provide a more comprehensive assessment of health than traditional measures like body mass index (BMI), offering insights into body fat percentage, muscle mass, and visceral fat levels.

**Tracking Progress:** By regularly monitoring changes in body composition over time, individuals can track the effectiveness of their diet and exercise interventions and adjust their strategies accordingly.

**Risk Stratification:** Abnormalities in body composition, such as excess visceral fat or low muscle mass, are associated with an increased risk of metabolic disorders and chronic diseases. Body composition analysis can help identify individuals at higher risk and guide targeted interventions to improve health outcomes.

## Functional Medicine Testing

Functional medicine testing involves a comprehensive evaluation of an individual's physiological function, including hormonal balance, nutrient status, and metabolic markers. These tests often include assessments of biomarkers such as cortisol levels, thyroid hormones, vitamin D levels, and inflammatory markers.

**Benefits:**

**Holistic Assessment:** Functional medicine testing provides a holistic view of an individual's health, allowing for a deeper understanding of underlying imbalances or dysfunctions that may contribute to metabolic issues.

**Personalized Treatment Plans:** Based on the results of functional medicine testing, healthcare providers can develop personalized treatment plans tailored to address specific imbalances or deficiencies identified in the individual's physiology.

**Preventive Care:** By detecting imbalances or dysfunctions in the body at an early stage, functional medicine testing enables proactive interventions to prevent the development of chronic diseases and optimize overall health and well-being.

## Practical Guide to Self-Monitoring

Embarking on a journey to optimize metabolic health requires a proactive approach to self-monitoring. By regularly tracking key metrics and making data-driven decisions, individuals can gain valuable insights into their health status and progress towards their wellness goals. This practical guide provides actionable steps for implementing self-monitoring practices and leveraging health technology to support metabolic health optimization.

### 1. Establish Baseline Metrics

Before diving into self-monitoring, it's essential to establish baseline metrics to track progress effectively. Schedule a comprehensive health assessment with your healthcare provider to measure key biomarkers such as blood glucose levels, lipid profile, body composition, and inflammatory markers. These baseline measurements will serve as a reference point for tracking changes over time.

### 2. Choose Appropriate Monitoring Tools

Selecting the right monitoring tools is crucial for accurate and convenient self-monitoring. Consider investing in wearable devices, such as smartwatches or fitness trackers, to track daily activity levels, sleep patterns, and heart rate variability. For individuals with diabetes or insulin resistance, continuous glucose monitors (CGMs) provide real-time data on blood glucose levels, enabling proactive management of dietary choices and insulin therapy.

## 3. Develop a Monitoring Routine

Establish a regular monitoring routine to track key metrics consistently. Set aside dedicated time each day or week to record data from your monitoring devices and update your health tracking app or journal. Consistency is key to identifying patterns, trends, and deviations from your baseline metrics, allowing for timely interventions when necessary.

## 4. Track Relevant Metrics

Focus on tracking metrics that are relevant to your metabolic health goals and priorities. For example, if weight management is a primary concern, monitor body weight, body fat percentage, and waist circumference regularly. If you're managing blood glucose levels, track fasting blood glucose readings, postprandial glucose levels, and HbA1c values diligently.

## 5. Interpret and Analyze Data

Once you've collected sufficient data, take the time to interpret and analyze the information to gain meaningful insights into your health status and progress. Look for patterns, trends, and correlations between different metrics, and consider how lifestyle factors such as diet, exercise, sleep, and stress may be influencing your health outcomes.

## 6. Set SMART Goals

Based on your analysis of the data, set specific, measurable, achievable, relevant, and time-bound (SMART) goals to guide your health and wellness journey. Whether it's achieving target blood glucose levels, reducing body fat percentage, or improving cardiovascular fitness, SMART goals provide a clear roadmap for success and help maintain motivation and accountability.

## 7. Adjust and Iterate

Regularly review your monitoring data and reassess your goals to ensure they remain aligned with your evolving health needs and priorities. Be prepared to adjust your monitoring routine, tracking metrics, or intervention strategies as needed based on feedback from your monitoring data and progress towards your goals.

## 8. Seek Professional Guidance

While self-monitoring is a valuable tool for optimizing metabolic health, it's essential to consult with qualified healthcare professionals for personalized guidance and support. Share your monitoring data with your healthcare provider during routine check-ups or virtual consultations, and collaborate on

developing tailored interventions and treatment plans
to address any identified issues or concerns.

CHAPTER 3: NUTRITION:
SIMPLIFYING DIETARY CHOICES

# CHAPTER 3: NUTRITION: SIMPLIFYING DIETARY CHOICES

**Eating for Energy: Food Principles for Optimal Health**

## Demystifying Dietary Philosophies

In the realm of nutrition, a myriad of dietary philosophies abound, each promising to unlock the secrets to optimal health and longevity. From low-carb to plant-based, ketogenic to Mediterranean, the plethora of dietary approaches can be overwhelming and confusing. Demystifying these dietary philosophies is essential for individuals seeking clarity on how to nourish their bodies for metabolic health and overall well-being. This chapter explores common dietary philosophies, their underlying principles, and their potential impact on metabolic function.

**Low-Carb/Ketogenic Diet**

**Principles:**

**Carbohydrate Restriction:** Low-carb and ketogenic diets emphasize minimizing carbohydrate intake to induce ketosis, a metabolic state where the body burns fat for fuel instead of carbohydrates.

High Fat, Moderate Protein: These diets typically include a higher intake of healthy fats, such as avocados, nuts, seeds, and olive oil, and moderate amounts of protein from sources like meat, fish, and eggs.

**Potential Impact on Metabolic Function:**

**Improved Insulin Sensitivity:** By reducing carbohydrate intake, low-carb and ketogenic diets may enhance insulin sensitivity and stabilize blood glucose levels, making them potentially beneficial for individuals with insulin resistance or type 2 diabetes.

**Weight Loss:** Ketogenic diets have been shown to promote weight loss by promoting fat burning and reducing appetite, although long-term adherence may vary.

**Plant-Based/Vegetarian/Vegan Diet**

**Principles:**

**Emphasis on Plant Foods:** Plant-based diets prioritize whole, minimally processed plant foods, including fruits, vegetables, grains, legumes, nuts, and seeds, while minimizing or excluding animal products.

**Variety and Balance:** A well-planned plant-based diet provides a diverse array of nutrients, including fiber, vitamins, minerals, and phytonutrients, while reducing the intake of saturated fat and cholesterol found in animal products.

**Potential Impact on Metabolic Function:**

**Heart Health:** Plant-based diets are associated with lower risk factors for cardiovascular disease, including reduced cholesterol levels, blood pressure, and inflammation.

**Blood Sugar Control:** The high fiber content of plant-based diets may help stabilize blood glucose levels and improve insulin sensitivity, potentially reducing the risk of type 2 diabetes.

**Mediterranean Diet**

**Principles:**

**Based on Traditional Mediterranean Eating Patterns**: The Mediterranean diet emphasizes whole, minimally processed foods commonly consumed in Mediterranean countries, including fruits, vegetables, whole grains, olive oil, fish, nuts, and legumes.

**Moderate Consumption of Animal Products:** While not strictly vegetarian, the Mediterranean diet includes moderate amounts of fish, poultry, dairy, and occasional red meat, typically consumed in smaller portions and less frequently than plant foods.

**Potential Impact on Metabolic Function:**

**Heart Health:** The Mediterranean diet is renowned for its cardiovascular benefits, including reduced risk of heart disease, stroke, and mortality. Its emphasis on olive oil, fish, nuts, and fiber-rich foods contributes to favorable lipid profiles and blood pressure levels.

**Anti-Inflammatory Effects:** The abundance of fruits, vegetables, and omega-3 fatty acids in the Mediterranean diet may help reduce inflammation, a key driver of metabolic dysfunction and chronic disease.

**Intermittent Fasting**

**Principles:**

**Periods of Fasting and Feeding:** Intermittent fasting involves cycling between periods of eating and fasting, with various fasting protocols ranging from daily time-restricted feeding (e.g., 16/8 method) to alternate-day fasting or periodic extended fasts.

**Metabolic Switch:** Fasting periods trigger metabolic adaptations that promote fat burning, ketone production, cellular repair, and autophagy (cellular cleansing).

**Potential Impact on Metabolic Function:**

**Weight Management:** Intermittent fasting can facilitate weight loss by reducing calorie intake and increasing fat oxidation, although individual responses may vary.

**Metabolic Flexibility:** Regular fasting may enhance metabolic flexibility, the body's ability to switch between burning glucose and fat for fuel, potentially improving insulin sensitivity and metabolic health.

Navigating the vast landscape of dietary advice can be daunting, but at the core of any healthy eating plan are fundamental principles that stand the test of time. These six lifelong food principles provide a solid foundation for nourishing your body, supporting metabolic health, and promoting overall well-being. Embracing these principles can help you make informed choices about the foods you consume, leading to sustainable habits that promote vitality and longevity.

## 1. Prioritize Whole, Unprocessed Foods

Whole, unprocessed foods are the cornerstone of a healthy diet, providing essential nutrients in their most natural form. Choose whole grains, fruits, vegetables, legumes, nuts, seeds, and minimally processed animal products over highly refined and processed foods. Whole foods are rich in vitamins, minerals, fiber, and phytonutrients, supporting optimal metabolic function and reducing the risk of chronic diseases.

## 2. Emphasize Dietary Diversity

Variety is key to a well-rounded diet that meets your body's nutritional needs. Aim to include a wide range of foods from all food groups in your meals and snacks. Each food group offers unique nutrients and health benefits, so diversifying your diet ensures you receive a broad spectrum of essential nutrients, antioxidants, and bioactive compounds that promote metabolic health and support overall vitality.

## 3. Prioritize Plant-Based Foods

Plant-based foods should form the foundation of your diet, providing the majority of your daily calorie intake. Fruits, vegetables, whole grains, legumes, nuts, and seeds are rich sources of fiber, antioxidants, vitamins, and minerals that support metabolic health, reduce inflammation, and lower the risk of chronic diseases. Aim to fill your plate with colorful, plant-based foods at every meal to maximize nutrient intake and promote well-being.

## 4. Choose Healthy Fats

Healthy fats play a crucial role in supporting metabolic health and overall well-being. Opt for sources of unsaturated fats, such as avocados, nuts, seeds, olive oil, and fatty fish, which provide essential omega-3 and omega-6 fatty acids that support heart health, brain function, and inflammation control. Limit your intake of saturated and trans fats found in processed foods, fried foods, and fatty meats, as they can contribute to metabolic dysfunction and cardiovascular disease risk.

## 5. Mindful Eating and Portion Control

Practicing mindful eating and portion control is essential for maintaining a healthy weight and optimizing metabolic function. Pay attention to hunger and fullness cues, eat slowly, and savor each bite to enhance satisfaction and reduce overeating. Use smaller plates and utensils, and be mindful of portion sizes to avoid excessive calorie intake. By listening to your body's hunger and satiety signals, you can cultivate a healthy relationship with food and support metabolic balance.

## 6. Stay Hydrated and Limit Sugary Beverages

Hydration is vital for metabolic health and overall well-being. Aim to drink plenty of water throughout the day to maintain proper hydration levels and support cellular function. Limit your intake of sugary beverages such as soda, fruit juices, and sweetened beverages, as they provide empty calories and contribute to insulin resistance, weight gain, and metabolic dysfunction. Opt for water, herbal teas, or infused water with fresh fruits and herbs as healthier alternatives to sugary drinks.

## Personalized Nutrition Plans for Every Lifestyle

In today's diverse and dynamic world, no single nutrition plan fits all. The concept of personalised nutrition acknowledges that every person has different nutritional requirements, preferences, and objectives depending on their age, gender, heredity, degree of exercise, health, and cultural background. By tailoring nutrition plans to accommodate these individual differences, personalized nutrition offers a more effective and sustainable approach to optimizing health and well-being. This chapter explores the concept of personalized nutrition and provides guidance on creating personalized nutrition plans to suit various lifestyles.

## Understanding Personalized Nutrition

Personalized nutrition goes beyond one-size-fits-all dietary recommendations and takes into account the individual's biological makeup, lifestyle factors, and personal preferences. It leverages advancements in science and technology, such as genetic testing, microbiome analysis, and wearable devices, to gather data and insights that inform personalized dietary recommendations. By considering factors such as nutrient needs, food sensitivities, metabolic status, and behavioral patterns, personalized nutrition aims to create tailored nutrition plans that optimize health outcomes and support long-term adherence.

## Factors Influencing Personalized Nutrition Plans

**Genetics:** Genetic variations influence how individuals metabolize nutrients and respond to dietary components. Genetic testing can identify genetic predispositions related to nutrient metabolism, food intolerances, and disease risk, guiding personalized dietary recommendations.

**Metabolic Health:** Individuals with conditions such as diabetes, obesity, or metabolic syndrome may require specific dietary interventions to manage their condition and improve metabolic health. Personalized nutrition plans can address individual metabolic needs, such as blood sugar control, insulin sensitivity, and lipid profiles.

**Lifestyle Factors:** Lifestyle factors, including activity level, stress levels, sleep patterns, and social dynamics, play a significant role in shaping dietary habits and nutritional requirements. Personalized nutrition plans take into account these lifestyle factors to develop strategies that support overall well-being and enhance adherence to dietary recommendations.

**Food Preferences and Culture:** Personal food preferences, cultural traditions, and culinary habits greatly influence dietary choices and eating behaviors. Personalized nutrition plans accommodate these preferences and cultural considerations to ensure dietary recommendations are enjoyable, satisfying, and culturally appropriate.

**Dietary Restrictions and Allergies:** Individuals with dietary restrictions, food allergies, or intolerances require personalized nutrition plans that address their specific dietary needs while ensuring adequate nutrient intake and variety. Personalized nutrition plans can offer alternative food options and substitutes to accommodate these dietary restrictions.

**Creating Personalized Nutrition Plans**

**Assessment and Data Collection:** Conduct a comprehensive assessment of the individual's health status, dietary habits, lifestyle factors, and goals. Gather data from sources such as health history questionnaires, food diaries, genetic testing, biomarker analysis, and wearable device data to inform personalized dietary recommendations.

**Identify Nutritional Needs:** Identify the individual's nutritional needs based on factors such as age, gender, activity level, metabolic status, and health goals. Consider specific nutrient requirements, such as protein, carbohydrates, fats, vitamins, minerals, and phytonutrients, to develop personalized nutrition plans that meet these needs.

**Tailor Dietary Recommendations:** Tailor dietary recommendations to align with the individual's nutritional needs, preferences, and goals. Consider factors such as macronutrient distribution, meal timing, portion sizes, food choices, and cooking methods to create personalized nutrition plans that are practical, enjoyable, and sustainable.

**Monitor Progress and Adjustments:** Continuously monitor the individual's progress and make adjustments to the personalized nutrition plan as needed. Regularly assess changes in health status, dietary adherence, metabolic markers, and behavioral patterns to optimize nutrition interventions and support long-term success.

**Personalized Nutrition Plans for Different Lifestyles**

**Busy Professionals:** For individuals with hectic schedules, personalized nutrition plans may focus on convenient and portable meal options, batch cooking and meal prep strategies, and time-saving cooking techniques to ensure nutritious eating habits despite busy lifestyles.

**Athletes and Fitness Enthusiasts:** Personalized nutrition plans for athletes and fitness enthusiasts may emphasize optimal fueling strategies for performance, including pre- and post-workout nutrition, hydration strategies, macronutrient timing, and supplementation to support energy levels, recovery, and muscle growth.

**Vegetarians and Vegans:** Personalized nutrition plans for vegetarians and vegans focus on ensuring adequate intake of essential nutrients such as protein, iron, calcium, vitamin B12, and omega-3 fatty acids from plant-based sources while optimizing dietary diversity and variety.

**Individuals with Chronic Conditions:** For individuals with chronic conditions such as diabetes, cardiovascular disease, or gastrointestinal disorders, personalized nutrition plans may incorporate dietary interventions tailored to manage specific symptoms, optimize metabolic health, and reduce disease risk factors.

**Cultural and Ethnic Considerations:** Personalized nutrition plans take into account cultural and ethnic food preferences and traditions, offering dietary recommendations that respect cultural norms while promoting health and well-being.

# CHAPTER 4: LIFESTYLE STRATEGIES FOR METABOLIC OPTIMIZATION

**Integrating Sleep, Movement, and Environmental Factors**

**The Role of Sleep and Circadian Rhythm in Metabolism**

Sleep is a fundamental physiological process that plays a crucial role in regulating metabolism, energy balance, and overall health. The circadian rhythm, often referred to as the body's internal clock, orchestrates a wide range of metabolic processes that occur in synchrony with the daily cycles of light and darkness. Disruptions to sleep patterns and circadian rhythm can have profound effects on metabolic health, increasing the risk of obesity, insulin resistance, diabetes, cardiovascular disease, and other metabolic disorders. Understanding the intricate interplay between sleep, circadian rhythm, and metabolism is essential for promoting optimal health and well-being.

## 1. Sleep Architecture and Metabolic Regulation

**Sleep Stages:**

**Non-Rapid Eye Movement (NREM) Sleep:** Divided into three stages (N1, N2, N3), characterized by progressively deeper sleep, slowed brain waves, and reduced muscle activity. NREM sleep is associated with restorative functions, including tissue repair, growth hormone secretion, and immune function.

**Rapid Eye Movement (REM) Sleep:** Marked by rapid eye movements, increased brain activity, and vivid dreaming. Memory consolidation, emotional control, and cognitive function all depend on REM sleep.

**Hormonal Regulation:**

**Leptin and Ghrelin:** Sleep deprivation disrupts the balance of hunger-regulating hormones, increasing levels of ghrelin (appetite-stimulating hormone) and decreasing levels of leptin (appetite-suppressing hormone), leading to increased appetite and food intake.

**Insulin Sensitivity:** Inadequate sleep impairs insulin sensitivity, disrupts glucose metabolism, and promotes insulin resistance, increasing the risk of type 2 diabetes and obesity.

**Cortisol:** Sleep deprivation elevates cortisol levels, a stress hormone associated with increased appetite, abdominal fat deposition, and metabolic dysfunction.

**Energy Balance:**

**Caloric Intake and Expenditure:** Sleep influences energy balance by modulating appetite, food cravings, and energy expenditure. Sleep deprivation alters food preferences towards high-calorie, carbohydrate-rich foods and reduces physical activity levels, contributing to weight gain and obesity.

## 2. Circadian Rhythm and Metabolic Regulation

**Circadian Clock:**

**Central and Peripheral Clocks:** The circadian rhythm is governed by a master clock located in the suprachiasmatic nucleus (SCN) of the hypothalamus, as well as peripheral clocks located in various tissues and organs throughout the body. These clocks synchronize physiological processes with the 24-hour light-dark cycle.

**Gene Expression:** Circadian clocks regulate the expression of genes involved in metabolism, including those responsible for nutrient uptake, energy production, glucose and lipid metabolism, and mitochondrial function.

**Metabolic Processes:**

**Glucose Homeostasis:** Circadian rhythms influence glucose homeostasis by regulating insulin secretion, glucose uptake, and gluconeogenesis. Disruptions to circadian rhythm disrupt glucose metabolism, leading to impaired fasting glucose levels and insulin resistance.

**Lipid Metabolism:** Circadian clocks regulate lipid metabolism by modulating lipid synthesis, storage, and oxidation. Dysregulation of circadian rhythm disrupts lipid metabolism, contributing to dyslipidemia and increased risk of cardiovascular disease.

**Energy Expenditure:** Circadian clocks influence energy expenditure through the regulation of metabolic rate, thermogenesis, and physical activity levels. Disruptions to circadian rhythm can lead to reduced energy expenditure and metabolic inefficiency.

### 3. Strategies for Promoting Healthy Sleep and Circadian Rhythm

**Sleep Hygiene Practices:**

**Consistent Sleep pattern:** Even on weekends, keep a regular sleep and wake pattern by retiring to bed and getting up at the same times every day.

**Sleep Environment:** Create a comfortable sleep environment that is dark, quiet, and conducive to sleep. Use blackout curtains, white noise machines, and comfortable bedding to optimize sleep quality.

**Limit Stimulants:** Avoid stimulants such as caffeine, nicotine, and alcohol close to bedtime, as they can interfere with sleep quality and disrupt circadian rhythm.

**Circadian Rhythm Synchronization:**

**Exposure to Natural Light:** Spend time outdoors during daylight hours to synchronize circadian rhythm with the natural light-dark cycle. Diminish exposure to artificial light, especially blue light from electronic devices, in the evening to promote melatonin production and prepare the body for sleep.

**Meal Timing:** Align meal timing with natural circadian rhythms by consuming larger meals earlier in the day and avoiding heavy meals close to bedtime. This helps regulate metabolism and supports healthy digestion.

**Stress Management and Relaxation Techniques:**

**Mindfulness Meditation:** Practice mindfulness meditation, deep breathing exercises, or progressive muscle relaxation techniques to reduce stress and promote relaxation before bedtime.

**Physical Activity:** Engage in regular physical activity, but avoid vigorous exercise close to bedtime, as it can increase alertness and delay sleep onset. Moderate exercise earlier in the day can help promote better sleep quality.

## Exercise Redefined: Incorporating Movement into Daily Life

In the modern era where sedentary lifestyles are prevalent, redefining exercise to incorporate movement into daily life is essential for promoting physical activity, improving health outcomes, and enhancing overall well-being. Rather than viewing exercise as a separate, structured activity confined to gym sessions or workout routines, embracing movement as an integral part of daily life encourages individuals to adopt a more active lifestyle that supports health and vitality. This chapter explores the concept of redefining exercise, practical strategies for incorporating movement into daily life, and the numerous health benefits associated with an active lifestyle.

## Understanding Exercise Redefined

Exercise redefined shifts the focus from traditional, structured exercise routines to incorporating movement into everyday activities, tasks, and routines. It emphasizes the importance of frequent, low-intensity movement throughout the day, rather than relying solely on intermittent bouts of vigorous exercise. By integrating movement into daily life, individuals can accumulate physical activity gradually, improve overall fitness levels, and reap the health benefits associated with an active lifestyle.

## Practical Strategies for Incorporating Movement

### 1. Active Commuting:

Walking or Biking: Opt for walking or biking as a mode of transportation whenever possible, whether it's commuting to work, running errands, or traveling short distances. This not only adds physical activity to your day but also reduces carbon emissions and supports environmental sustainability.

## 2. Active Workstations:

Standing Desk: Invest in a standing desk or adjustable workstation that allows you to alternate between sitting and standing throughout the day. Incorporate periodic standing breaks, gentle stretching, or short walks to break up prolonged periods of sitting and promote circulation.

## 3. Household Chores and Tasks:

Multitasking Movement: Turn household chores and tasks into opportunities for movement by incorporating squats while doing laundry, lunges while vacuuming, or calf raises while washing dishes. This adds a functional aspect to exercise and makes it more manageable within busy schedules.

## 4. Incorporating Movement Breaks:

Microbreaks: Take short movement breaks every hour to stretch, stand, or walk around. Set reminders or use smartphone apps to prompt regular breaks and prevent prolonged sitting.

## 5. Active Leisure Activities:

Outdoor Recreation: Engage in outdoor leisure activities such as hiking, gardening, swimming, or playing sports with friends and family. These activities not only provide opportunities for movement but also offer mental and emotional benefits associated with nature and social interaction.

**Health Benefits of Incorporating Movement**

**1. Improved Physical Health:**

**Cardiovascular Health:** Regular movement supports cardiovascular health by reducing the risk of heart disease, hypertension, and stroke. Incorporating movement into daily life improves circulation, lowers blood pressure, and enhances cardiovascular function.

**Weight Management:** Incorporating movement throughout the day helps burn calories, increase metabolic rate, and support weight management efforts. It contributes to a more active lifestyle and aids in achieving and maintaining a healthy body weight.

**2. Enhanced Mental Well-Being:**

**Stress Reduction:** Movement has stress-relieving effects by promoting the release of endorphins, neurotransmitters that elevate mood and reduce feelings of stress and anxiety. Incorporating movement into daily life can help alleviate tension, improve mental clarity, and enhance overall well-being.

**Cognitive Function:** Regular physical activity, including movement-based activities, has been shown to enhance cognitive function, memory, and concentration. It promotes neuroplasticity, the brain's ability to adapt and reorganize in response to stimuli, leading to improved cognitive performance and mental acuity.

## 3. Increased Energy Levels:

**Combatting Fatigue:** Movement stimulates circulation, oxygenates tissues, and boosts energy levels by increasing blood flow and delivering nutrients and oxygen to cells. Incorporating movement breaks throughout the day can help combat fatigue, reduce feelings of lethargy, and promote alertness and vitality.

## 4. Enhanced Quality of Life:

**Functional Mobility:** Regular movement supports functional mobility by maintaining joint flexibility, muscle strength, and balance. It reduces the risk of falls, improves posture, and enhances overall physical function, leading to greater independence and autonomy in daily activities.

**Longevity:** Incorporating movement into daily life is associated with increased longevity and reduced risk of premature mortality. It promotes healthy aging by preserving physiological function, mitigating age-related declines, and supporting overall vitality and longevity.

## Harnessing the Benefits of Cold and Heat Exposure

Cold and heat exposure are two powerful modalities that have been utilized for centuries to promote health, enhance resilience, and optimize overall well-being. From traditional practices like cold water immersion and sauna bathing to modern therapies such as cryotherapy and heat therapy, harnessing the benefits of cold and heat exposure offers a range of physiological and psychological effects that support health and vitality. This chapter explores the mechanisms underlying cold and heat exposure, practical applications of these modalities, and the potential health benefits they provide.

**1. Cold Exposure:** Understanding the Mechanisms

**Thermogenesis and Metabolic Activation:**

**Brown Adipose Tissue (BAT):** Cold exposure stimulates the activation of brown adipose tissue, a specialized type of fat that generates heat through thermogenesis. BAT activation increases energy expenditure, improves insulin sensitivity, and may contribute to weight management.

**Adaptive Thermogenesis:** Prolonged exposure to cold triggers adaptive thermogenesis, a process that enhances the body's ability to generate heat and maintain core temperature. This metabolic adaptation improves cold tolerance and resilience to environmental stressors.

**Immune Modulation and Inflammation:**

**Cold Shock Response:** Cold exposure activates the body's cold shock response, triggering physiological changes that modulate immune function and inflammation. Cold-induced stress activates pathways involved in immune regulation, reducing inflammation and enhancing immune surveillance.

**Cold-Induced Hormesis:** Mild cold stress induces hormetic responses in the body, triggering adaptive changes that enhance resilience and resistance to oxidative stress, inflammation, and disease.

## 2. Heat Exposure: Exploring the Benefits

**Vasodilation and Circulation:**

**Heat Stress Response:** Heat exposure induces vasodilation and increases blood flow to the skin, facilitating heat dissipation and promoting circulation. Heat-induced vasodilation improves cardiovascular function, enhances nutrient delivery, and supports tissue repair and recovery.

**Sauna Therapy:** Sauna bathing promotes relaxation, detoxification, and cardiovascular conditioning by exposing the body to heat stress. Regular sauna use has been associated with reduced cardiovascular risk, improved endothelial function, and enhanced exercise performance.

## Heat Shock Proteins (HSPs) and Cellular Health:

HSP Induction: Heat exposure stimulates the production of heat shock proteins (HSPs), molecular chaperones that protect cells from stress and promote cellular repair and resilience. HSP induction enhances cellular detoxification, protein folding, and DNA repair mechanisms.

**Anti-Aging Effects:** Heat stress-induced HSPs exert anti-aging effects by preserving cellular integrity, enhancing mitochondrial function, and mitigating age-related declines in cellular function. Heat therapy may promote longevity and support healthy aging.

## 3. Practical Applications and Considerations

### Cold Exposure:

**Cold Water Immersion:** Cold water immersion, such as ice baths or cold showers, is a popular method for harnessing the benefits of cold exposure. Start with brief exposures and gradually increase duration and intensity to build tolerance and avoid overexertion.

**Cryotherapy:** Cryotherapy involves exposing the body to extremely cold temperatures in specialized cryo-chambers or cryo-saunas. Cryotherapy sessions typically last a few minutes and may provide rapid recovery, pain relief, and performance enhancement benefits.

**Heat Exposure:**

**Sauna Bathing:** Regular sauna bathing sessions, lasting 15-20 minutes at temperatures of 160-200°F (70-95°C), offer numerous health benefits, including cardiovascular conditioning, relaxation, detoxification, and immune modulation. To avoid dehydration and excessive heat, stay hydrated and limit the length of your sauna sessions.

**Hot Yoga and Heat Therapy:** Hot yoga classes and heat therapy treatments, such as infrared sauna therapy, provide additional options for heat exposure. These practices promote flexibility, relaxation, and stress relief while enhancing circulation and detoxification.

## 4. Health Benefits and Considerations

**Overall Health Benefits:**

**Improved Circulation:** Both cold and heat exposure promote circulation, enhance nutrient delivery, and support tissue repair and recovery.

**Stress Reduction:** Cold and heat exposure have stress-reducing effects, promoting relaxation, reducing inflammation, and enhancing resilience to environmental stressors.

**Metabolic Activation:** Cold exposure activates thermogenic pathways, while heat exposure induces heat shock proteins, leading to metabolic activation and improved energy metabolism.

## Considerations and Precautions:

**Individual Variability:** Responses to cold and heat exposure vary among individuals, so it's essential to start gradually and listen to your body's cues. Consult with a healthcare professional before initiating cold or heat exposure practices, especially if you have underlying health conditions or concerns.

**Hydration and Rest:** Stay hydrated and well-rested before and after cold or heat exposure sessions to support recovery and minimize potential side effects. Pay attention to signs of dehydration, overheating, or discomfort and adjust exposure accordingly.

# CHAPTER 5: NAVIGATING THE MEDICAL SYSTEM FOR BETTER HEALTH

## Getting What You Need from Healthcare Providers

### Effective Communication with Doctors: A Guide to Advocating for Your Health

Effective communication with doctors is essential for building trust, fostering collaboration, and ensuring that your healthcare needs are met. Whether you're seeking guidance for a specific health concern, discussing treatment options, or navigating complex medical decisions, clear and open communication with your healthcare provider is paramount. This chapter provides practical tips and strategies for effectively communicating with doctors, advocating for your health, and maximizing the quality of care you receive.

## 1. Prepare for Your Appointment

**Gather Information:**

**Medical History:** Compile a comprehensive medical history, including past illnesses, surgeries, medications, and allergies. Provide relevant medical records or test results to your doctor to facilitate informed decision-making.

**Symptom Diary:** Keep a record of symptoms, including their onset, duration, severity, and any factors that worsen or alleviate them. This information can help your doctor make an accurate diagnosis and develop an appropriate treatment plan.

**Questions and Concerns:** Prepare a list of questions and concerns you want to discuss during your appointment. Prioritize your concerns to ensure that important topics are addressed within the allotted time.

## 2. Establish Open Communication

**Build Rapport:**

**Establish Trust:** Foster a trusting relationship with your doctor by being open, honest, and respectful. Share relevant information about your health, lifestyle, and preferences to facilitate personalized care.

**Active Listening:** Listen attentively to your doctor's explanations, instructions, and recommendations. Ask clarifying questions if you don't understand something, and seek additional information or resources as needed.

**Be Transparent:**

**Share Concerns:** Voice any concerns or uncertainties you have about your health, treatment options, or prognosis. Expressing your feelings and preferences openly allows your doctor to address them effectively and tailor care to your individual needs.

**Provide Feedback:** Offer feedback about your experiences with healthcare services, including communication, coordination of care, and access to resources. Constructive feedback helps identify areas for improvement and enhances the quality of care provided.

## 3. Advocate for Your Health

**Be Proactive:**

**Ask Questions:** Don't hesitate to ask questions or seek clarification about medical terms, procedures, or treatment plans. Empower yourself with knowledge and actively participate in decision-making regarding your health.

**Seek Second Opinions:** If you have reservations about a diagnosis or treatment plan, consider seeking a second opinion from another qualified healthcare provider. Multiple perspectives can provide valuable insights and options for consideration.

**Assert Your Needs:**

**Express Preferences:** Communicate your preferences regarding treatment options, care settings, and involvement in decision-making. Your doctor should respect your autonomy and involve you in decisions that affect your health and well-being.

**Clarify Expectations:** Clearly communicate your expectations regarding communication frequency, follow-up appointments, and access to medical records or test results. Establishing clear expectations promotes accountability and ensures continuity of care.

### 4. Follow Up and Stay Engaged

**Follow Through:**

**Follow Treatment Plans:** Adhere to treatment plans, medication regimens, and lifestyle recommendations prescribed by your doctor. If you encounter challenges or side effects, discuss them with your doctor promptly to explore alternative options.

**Attend Follow-Up Appointments:** Schedule and attend follow-up appointments as recommended by your doctor to monitor progress, adjust treatment as needed, and address any new concerns or developments.

**Stay Informed:**

**Stay Educated:** Stay informed about your health condition, treatment options, and available resources through reputable sources such as medical journals, patient advocacy organizations, and trusted healthcare websites. Learning gives you the ability to take an active role in your care and make wise decisions.

**Engage in Shared Decision-Making:** Collaborate with your doctor to make decisions that align with your values, preferences, and goals. Participate in shared decision-making discussions by weighing the benefits, risks, and trade-offs of different treatment options.

## Essential Medical Tests and When to Request Them

Regular medical tests play a crucial role in maintaining health, detecting potential health issues early, and guiding appropriate interventions. However, navigating the landscape of medical tests can be overwhelming, with numerous options available for different health concerns and risk factors. Understanding which medical tests are essential and when to request them is essential for optimizing preventive care and promoting overall well-being. This chapter provides an overview of essential medical tests across various health domains and guidance on when to request them based on individual health needs and risk factors.

### 1. General Health Screenings

**Blood Pressure Measurement:**

**When to Request:** Regular blood pressure measurements are recommended for adults of all ages, especially those with risk factors such as hypertension, heart disease, diabetes, or a family history of high blood pressure.

**Frequency:** Blood pressure should be checked at least once every two years for adults with normal blood pressure readings. People who have high blood pressure or other risk factors might need to be monitored more frequently.

### Lipid Profile (Cholesterol Test):

**When to Request:** A lipid profile is recommended for adults aged 20 and older, particularly those with risk factors for cardiovascular disease, such as obesity, diabetes, high blood pressure, or a family history of heart disease.

**Frequency:** A lipid profile is typically recommended every four to six years for adults with normal cholesterol levels. Individuals with elevated cholesterol levels or other risk factors may require more frequent testing.

### Blood Glucose Test (Blood Sugar Test):

**When to Request:** Blood glucose testing is recommended for individuals with risk factors for diabetes, such as obesity, sedentary lifestyle, family history of diabetes, or gestational diabetes during pregnancy.

**Frequency:** Screening for diabetes is typically recommended every three years for adults aged 45 and older, or earlier and more frequently for those with risk factors.

## 2. Cancer Screenings

### Breast Cancer Screening (Mammogram):

**When to Request:** Mammograms are recommended for women aged 50 to 74 years for routine breast cancer screening. Women with a family history of breast cancer or other risk factors may start screening earlier and undergo more frequent testing.

**Frequency:** Mammograms are typically performed every two years for women within the recommended screening age range.

### Colorectal Cancer Screening (Colonoscopy or Fecal Occult Blood Test):

**When to Request:** Colorectal cancer screening is recommended for adults aged 45 to 75 years, with earlier or more frequent testing for individuals with risk factors such as family history of colorectal cancer, personal history of inflammatory bowel disease, or certain genetic syndromes.

**Frequency:** Screening methods may vary based on individual risk factors and preferences, with options including colonoscopy every 10 years, fecal occult blood test (FOBT) every year, or other stool-based tests.

## Pap or HPV tests for the screening of cervical cancer:

**When to Request:** Cervical cancer screening is recommended for individuals with a cervix aged 21 to 65 years, with earlier or more frequent testing for those with risk factors such as human papillomavirus (HPV) infection, previous abnormal Pap test results, or immunosuppression.

**Frequency:** Pap tests are typically performed every three years for individuals aged 21 to 29 years, while co-testing with Pap and HPV tests every five years is recommended for individuals aged 30 to 65 years.

## 3. Other Essential Tests

### Bone Density Test (DXA Scan):

**When to Request:** Bone density testing is recommended for postmenopausal women aged 65 and older, or earlier for those with risk factors such as history of fractures, family history of osteoporosis, or long-term use of certain medications.

**Frequency:** Testing frequency may vary based on individual risk factors and results, with repeat testing recommended every one to two years as needed.

### The Basic Metabolic Panel (BMP) or Comprehensive Metabolic Panel (CMP):

**When to Request:** A comprehensive metabolic panel (CMP) or basic metabolic panel (BMP) may be ordered as part of routine health assessments or to evaluate specific symptoms or health conditions, such as kidney or liver function, electrolyte imbalances, or metabolic disorders.

**Frequency:** Testing frequency depends on individual health status and medical history, with repeat testing as needed to monitor changes or assess treatment effectiveness.

## Advocating for Your Health: Tips and Resources

Advocating for your health is a vital aspect of navigating the healthcare system, ensuring personalized care, and achieving optimal health outcomes. Whether you're managing a chronic condition, undergoing treatment for a health issue, or seeking preventive care, being an effective advocate empowers you to communicate your needs, make informed decisions, and collaborate with healthcare providers to achieve your health goals. This chapter provides practical tips and valuable resources to help you advocate for your health effectively and navigate the complexities of healthcare delivery.

### 1. Educate Yourself

**Research Your Health Condition:**

**Understand Your Diagnosis:** Take the time to research your health condition, including causes, symptoms, treatment options, and prognosis. Knowledge empowers you to ask informed questions, participate in decision-making, and advocate for appropriate care.

**Stay Updated:** Keep abreast of the latest developments in research, treatment options, and best practices related to your health condition. Reputable sources such as medical journals, patient advocacy organizations, and trusted healthcare websites can provide valuable information.

## 2. Communicate Effectively

**Build a Partnership with Your Healthcare Team:**

**Establish Open Communication:** Foster a collaborative relationship with your healthcare providers based on trust, mutual respect, and open communication. Share your concerns, preferences, and goals to ensure that your care aligns with your individual needs and values.

**Ask Questions:** Don't hesitate to ask questions or seek clarification about your health condition, treatment options, medications, or test results. Effective communication facilitates shared decision-making and enhances the quality of care provided.

## 3. Be Proactive

**Take Charge of Your Health:**

**Participate in Decision-Making:** Actively participate in decision-making regarding your health by weighing the benefits, risks, and alternatives of different treatment options. Your input is valuable in shaping your care plan and ensuring that it aligns with your preferences and priorities.

**Seek Second Opinions:** If you have doubts or uncertainties about a diagnosis or treatment plan, consider seeking a second opinion from another qualified healthcare provider. Multiple perspectives can provide valuable insights and options for consideration.

## 4. Know Your Rights

**Understand Your Healthcare Rights:**

**Patient Rights:** Familiarize yourself with your rights as a patient, including the right to informed consent, privacy, confidentiality, and access to your medical records. Asserting your rights empowers you to advocate for respectful and patient-centered care.

**Health Insurance Coverage:** Understand your health insurance coverage, including benefits, limitations, co-pays, deductibles, and out-of-pocket costs. Knowing your coverage helps you make informed decisions about healthcare services and financial responsibilities.

## 5. Access Support and Resources

**Seek Support Networks:**

**Patient Advocacy Organizations:** Connect with patient advocacy organizations and support groups dedicated to your specific health condition. These organizations offer valuable resources, educational materials, peer support, and advocacy opportunities for individuals and families affected by the condition.

**Healthcare Navigation Services:** Utilize healthcare navigation services offered by hospitals, clinics, or community organizations to access guidance, assistance, and resources for navigating the healthcare system and coordinating care.

**Empowering Your Health Journey**

**Recap of Key Concepts and Strategies**

Throughout this book, we've explored a wide range of concepts, strategies, and resources aimed at empowering you to optimize your health, advocate for your well-being, and navigate the complexities of the healthcare system. As we conclude, let's recap some of the key concepts and strategies discussed in this guide:

## 1. Understanding Your Health

Metabolic Function: Recognize the importance of metabolic function in overall health and well-being. Understand how cellular energy production, metabolic regulation, and biomarkers influence health outcomes.

## 2. Lifestyle Factors and Health Optimization

Nutrition: Embrace lifelong food principles and personalized nutrition plans to support metabolic health and well-being, regardless of dietary preferences.

Sleep and Circadian Rhythm: Prioritize sleep hygiene practices and circadian rhythm synchronization to support optimal metabolic function, cognitive performance, and overall health.

Physical Activity: Redefine exercise by incorporating movement into daily life, promoting physical activity, and enhancing resilience to disease and stress.

## 3. Holistic Health Approaches

Cold and Heat Exposure: Harness the benefits of cold and heat exposure to promote resilience, enhance metabolic function, and support overall well-being.

Effective Communication: Advocate for your health by building collaborative relationships with healthcare providers, communicating effectively, and participating in shared decision-making.

## 4. Preventive Care and Health Maintenance

Essential Medical Tests: Understand the importance of regular medical screenings for monitoring health, detecting potential issues early, and guiding preventive interventions.

Advocating for Your Health: Take an active role in your healthcare journey by educating yourself, communicating your needs, being proactive, knowing your rights, and accessing support and resources.

## 5. Empowerment and Self-Advocacy

Knowledge Empowerment: Empower yourself with knowledge about your health condition, treatment options, and available resources. Remain informed, pose inquiries, and, if required, obtain second viewpoints.

Patient-Centered Care: Advocate for patient-centered care by asserting your preferences, participating in decision-making, and collaborating with healthcare providers to achieve personalized health goals.

## Building a Sustainable Plan for Long-Term Wellness

Achieving long-term wellness involves more than just short-term fixes or temporary changes. It requires a comprehensive and sustainable approach that addresses all aspects of health—physical, mental, emotional, and social. Building a sustainable plan for long-term wellness involves adopting healthy habits, fostering resilience, and nurturing a supportive environment that promotes well-being. In this final chapter, we'll explore key principles and strategies for creating a sustainable plan for lifelong health and vitality.

## 1. Establish Clear Goals and Priorities

**Define Your Vision:**

**Reflect on Your Values:** Identify what matters most to you in life, whether it's spending time with loved ones, pursuing personal interests, or achieving professional goals. Align your health goals with your values to create a meaningful and purpose-driven wellness plan.

**Set Realistic Objectives:** Establish clear, achievable goals that reflect your priorities and aspirations. To stay motivated and monitor progress over time, break down more ambitious objectives into smaller, more doable tasks.

## 2. Adopt Healthy Lifestyle Habits

**Focus on Balanced Nutrition:**

**Eat Whole Foods:** Prioritize whole, nutrient-dense foods such as fruits, vegetables, lean proteins, whole grains, and healthy fats. Strive for balance and moderation in your diet, emphasizing variety and quality over restriction or deprivation.

**Keep Yourself Hydrated:** To promote digestion, hydration, and general health, sip copious amounts of water throughout the day.
 Limit sugary beverages and excessive caffeine intake, opting for water as your primary source of hydration.

**Prioritize Physical Activity:**

**Incorporate Movement:** Embrace a diverse range of physical activities that you enjoy, including walking, cycling, yoga, strength training, and outdoor recreation. The weekly goal should be at least 150 minutes of moderate-intensity activity or 75 minutes of vigorous-intensity exercise, plus two or more days of muscle-strengthening exercises.

**Cultivate Emotional Well-Being:**

**Practice Mindfulness:** Incorporate mindfulness techniques such as meditation, deep breathing, and progressive muscle relaxation into your daily routine to reduce stress, enhance resilience, and promote emotional well-being.

**Seek Support:** Build a strong support network of friends, family members, or mental health professionals who can provide emotional support, guidance, and encouragement during challenging times.

### 3. Foster Resilience and Adaptability

**Embrace Flexibility:**

**Be Adaptable:** Embrace change as a natural part of life and cultivate adaptability to navigate challenges and setbacks effectively. Focus on solutions, learn from experiences, and view obstacles as opportunities for growth and self-improvement.

**Practice Self-Compassion:** Be kind to yourself and practice self-compassion during times of difficulty or adversity. Show compassion and empathy for yourself as you would a friend going through a similar ordeal.

## 4. Create a Supportive Environment

### Surround Yourself with Positivity:

**Choose Supportive Relationships:** Surround yourself with positive, uplifting individuals who encourage and inspire you to pursue your goals and live your best life. Foster meaningful connections with people who share your values and support your well-being.

**Create Healthy Habits Together:** Involve friends, family members, or colleagues in your wellness journey by engaging in activities together, sharing healthy meals, and providing mutual support and accountability.

## 5. Practice Continuous Self-Care

### Prioritize Self-Care:

**Make Time for Yourself:** Schedule regular self-care activities that nourish your mind, body, and spirit. Whether it's reading a book, taking a long bath, or practicing a hobby you enjoy, prioritize activities that replenish your energy and promote relaxation.

**Listen to Your Body:** Pay attention to your body's signals and honor its needs for rest, nourishment, movement, and relaxation. Tune in to your intuition and practice intuitive self-care by responding to your body's cues with kindness and compassion.

Inspiring Stories of Success and Future Directions

As we conclude our journey towards optimizing health and well-being, it's essential to draw inspiration from real-life stories of individuals who have overcome challenges, transformed their lives, and embraced a path towards long-term wellness. These stories serve as reminders of the power of resilience, determination, and hope in the face of adversity. In this final chapter, we'll explore inspiring stories of success and look towards future directions in the pursuit of optimal health for all.

## 1. From Adversity to Triumph: Real-Life Success Stories

**Sarah's Journey to Wellness:**

Sarah struggled with obesity and related health issues for years, feeling trapped in a cycle of fad diets and yo-yo weight fluctuations. Determined to reclaim her health, she embarked on a journey of self-discovery, focusing on balanced nutrition, regular exercise, and mindfulness practices. Through perseverance and self-compassion, Sarah lost over 100 pounds, reversed her chronic conditions, and regained her vitality and zest for life. Today, she inspires others as a wellness coach, sharing her journey and empowering individuals to embrace sustainable lifestyle changes for long-term health and happiness.

## Mark's Transformation Through Resilience:

Mark faced a devastating diagnosis of type 2 diabetes and struggled with managing his condition and its complications. Despite setbacks and challenges, he refused to let diabetes define his life. With the support of his healthcare team and a commitment to self-care, Mark adopted a plant-based diet, incorporated regular exercise into his routine, and prioritized stress management techniques. Over time, his blood sugar levels stabilized, his energy levels soared, and he experienced a newfound sense of vitality and purpose. Mark now advocates for diabetes awareness and prevention, sharing his story of resilience and empowerment with others facing similar health challenges.

## 2. Future Directions in Health and Wellness

## Advancements in Personalized Medicine:

With rapid advancements in technology and medical research, the future of health and wellness is increasingly personalized and data-driven. From genomics and biomarker testing to wearable devices and digital health platforms, individuals have unprecedented access to tools and resources for optimizing their health and well-being. Personalized medicine holds the promise of tailored interventions, precision diagnostics, and targeted therapies that address the unique needs and preferences of each individual, revolutionizing healthcare delivery and improving health outcomes.

**Integrative Approaches to Holistic Health:**

The integration of conventional medicine with complementary and alternative therapies is gaining recognition as a holistic approach to health and wellness. From acupuncture and herbal medicine to yoga and meditation, integrative modalities offer diverse options for promoting physical, mental, and emotional well-being. By combining evidence-based practices with traditional healing modalities, integrative medicine addresses the whole person—body, mind, and spirit—and fosters a collaborative partnership between patients and healthcare providers.

www.ingramcontent.com/pod-product-compliance
Lightning Source LLC
Chambersburg PA
CBHW050817250726
48653CB00006B/2271